Einar,
It's all good!

Meditations
A Zottola Publishing Book

PUBLISHING HISTORY
Zottola Publishing paperback edition
published March 2004

All rights reserved
Copyright 2003 by Mike Strand

Cover design, interior illustrations and maps by Giovanna Fregni
Interior layout and design by Victor Raymond

Many thanks to
Dwight Dake for technical assistance

No part of this book may be reproduced or transmitted in any form or by any means, electronic or mechanical, including photocopying, recording, or by any information storage and retrieval system, without permission in writing from the publisher.

ISBN 0-9725880-5-1

Zottola Publishing, Inc.
www.zotpub.com

Printed in the United States of America
9 8 7 6 5 4 3 2 1

Meditations
on Brain Injury

by

Mike Strand

Mike Strand

Dedicated to
my loving wife Linda
without whose support
this would not have been possible
- *Mike Strand*

Meditations

Preface

Albert Einstein once said "Life is a gift and if we agree to accept it we must contribute in return. "

For the past four years, Mike Strand has been a contributing guest columnist for "HEADLINES" the Brain Injury Association of Minnesota's quarterly publication. We did not assign any topics to Mike; we simply wanted him to write within his area of expertise, life after brain injury from the inside out. To our great surprise and pleasure Mike excelled. Mike's column is the first thing many of us read. I hear regulary from individuals who have sustained a brain injury or their family members about the value of Mike's column. It renews the readers' desire to be the best they can be, it challenges them with a vision that their dreams are possible. Family members have commented about how they gained a deeper understanding of their loved ones' experiences because of Mike.

Part philosopher and part artist, Mike paints a vision for us that we all want to embrace. As the Executive Director for the Brain Injury Association of Minnesota I have learned much from my friends with brain injury and Mike has been one of the best teachers.

Having survived a traumatic brain injury 14 years ago Mike continually struggles to make the most of every asset he has. And he has many. By temperament, Mike is a remarkably serene man with an almost mystical sense of well being. Mike questions, yet is upbeat. He can be cynical, yet hopeful. He is serious, yet has a great sense of humor.

Mike Strand

Thanks to his continual contemplation many sage morsels of advice can be found throughout his writings.

The essays in this book offer many important insights about attitude. Mike often suggests ingenious strategies by which we can improve our lives. His writing help us to understand Mike, who he is, what he stands for and why. Mike's words reveal the constraints and opportunities he faces following his brain injury, and how they have shaped his dreams and aspirations.

Mike Strand inspires people to become better people. His writings create a sense of hope a sense that tomorrow can be a better place - timeless values that we can all strive for. Mike continually inspires people to take personal responsibility for making the best of their lives.

Tom Gode
Executive Director
Brain Injury Association of Minnesota

Meditations

An Introduction

These essays appeared in "Headlines," a newsletter from the Brain Injury Association of Minnesota. My column is entitled "Here and Now." All the essays are short for a reason. I feel that if I have something to say I should try to say it in as few words as possible. The reason for my laconic writing discipline is that I know it is very difficult for most brain injury victims to read. It is difficult to follow long passages and lengthy convoluted dialectics as well. My writing style is one of concision. Since everyone experiences things differently, and language is an imperfect communication medium at best, I attempt to stimulate further reflection on the part of my readers. A number of times I have been contacted by a reader who tells me that it was so great to finally have someone tell them that they are not alone, that they feel the same way, and then I learn that they drew an entirely different meaning from what I had intended. That is all right. In fact, that is better than all right, it means they drew more from my essay than what I had consciously put into it.

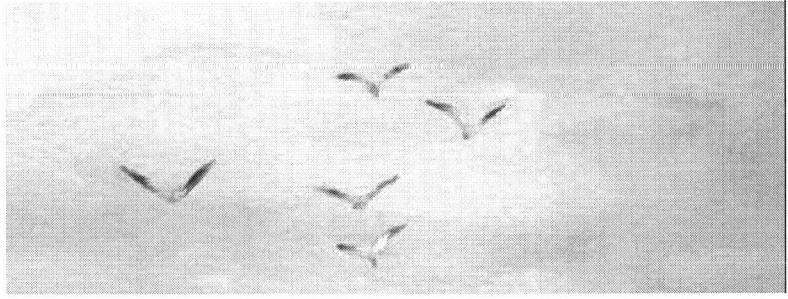

Mike Strand

I do have one wish. I don't want this book to be a "coffee table book." I want this book to be a "bathroom book." I want this book to be read, marked up, annotated. This is the perfect book to pick up whenever you have a spare moment to glance at a page or two.

Meditations

"Kharmatic Justice"

"Fred Cox!" I yelled as I lunged forward imitating the Minnesota Viking's star kicker's style and booted the red playground ball across the school yard to the dismay of my fellow class-mates who were trying to play Four-square with it. Oh for the halcyon days of my youth; I was ten at the time of my "Fred Cox" phase. Now I'm older and I've learned about personal responsibility and being accountable for my actions and the effect they have on others and the world I live in.

Likewise, I'm sure the kharmatic irony didn't occur to me during that split-second before Fred's boot, in the form of a gravel hauling semi-truck, slammed into the playground ball, now me and my Ford f-150 pick-up, and sent it hurtling seventy-five feet.

When the paramedics arrived they assumed I was just unconscious; then they took my pulse and blood pressure and were dismayed to discover that I probably would not make it to the hospital. I did make it to the hospital and ten days later I was drifting out of a coma and beginning my long (rest of my life) recovery.

I had to relearn to walk, talk, tie my shoes, read...everything. I was released from the hospital eight weeks later and returned to work after six months. It would be almost four years before I could work an eight-hour day.

Brain injury rehabilitation was the hardest thing I have ever done. Conversely, everything else now seems relatively easy. It doesn't matter if I'm training for a long distance run, sweating through a ninety-minute Bikram's hot yoga class, or trying to learn a foreign language in spite of the fact that I have almost no short term memory, or just getting dressed. It's all the same.

Mike Strand

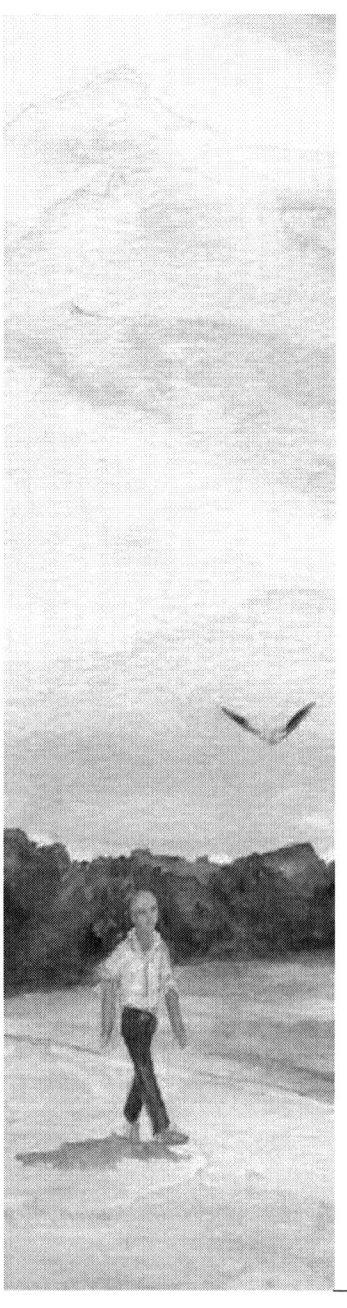

I've run ten mile races. I am a yoga instructor. I speak three languages besides English. I get dressed all by myself every day (unless we're going out, then my wife picks what I should wear). I'm not trying to brag, I'm merely underscoring how difficult recovering from brain injury is.

Getting the Most Out of Rehab

I normally write essays about recovery issues after one leaves the rehab environment, but first I'd like to focus on things I wish I had known while I was in rehab at the hospital.

Rehab felt a lot like elementary school to me. A lot of the subjects and tasks were the same, and of course, it was a very structured environment. I was asked to do a lot of things and I was not told why I needed to learn what I was doing; I was just supposed to accept the task on faith and try my best. Not surprisingly, I assumed a lot of the attitudes and habits that I had in school.

I didn't feel like I was doing these things for my own benefit. I felt like it was my job to please my rehab professionals. I felt like I was doing it for them. They were always making demands and offering praise if I obeyed. So I took a lot of short cuts and satisfied myself that whatever I had done was "good enough." I did what I figured was required to get by.

I knew the song and dance about how this was all for my benefit, but it didn't feel that way. If I had stepped back and thought about it, I would have admitted that I knew it was for my own good. On a day by day basis however, I felt like I was merely trying to accede to their demands.

Empty motions accomplish very little. What I really needed to do was explain to myself, *at every opportunity,* why I was doing the things I was doing, instead of just going through the motions. If I couldn't see the point to what I was doing then I should have asked.

Knowing why I am doing something is very important. It is the basis of motivation.

Mike Strand

I also believe in the power of the mind to heal. I think that if you tell yourself that you are going to learn how to do something for a reason or purpose, then your mind will obey. The mind is a powerful tool. Even the mind of a brain injured person. The brain is the wiring and the mind is the current that runs through the wires. The wiring may be damaged, but the current is still there.

Your brain is damaged, but you are still who you are. Your mind is still alive and thinking and feeling.

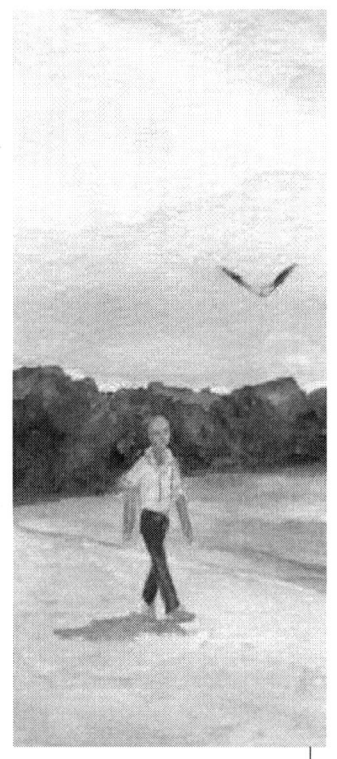

Sometimes I feel as if I'm trapped under the ice of a frozen lake. I'm still okay, but I can't get a message through. I pound and I pound on the ice, but the ice is thick and no one can hear me. It is cold, dark, and lonely. Above me there is light that I can not reach. I can see my friends and family walking on the ice above me, desperately looking for me and trying to get a message through to me. One by one I see them give up hope and walk away, shaking their heads and looking back every once in awhile, longing for me, feeling that I'm so close but fearing they will never see me again. This is the despair I feel. That picture beneath the frozen lake is the picture that's frozen in my mind.

That is why I struggle so hard to recover. That is why wellness isn't just a catchy phrase for me, but a moral imperative. To the extent that I have been successful, I wish to chronicle my achievements so that others can use my experiences to forge their own tools to chip through the ice.

It can be done.

Meditations

Making Sense of Brain Injury

This is an introduction on a series of three essays on self-improvement that I have found worked for me. I am sharing my twelve years of experience post-Traumatic Brain Injury (TBI) in the hopes that others may find bits and pieces that facilitate their own personal growth.

These are things that I wish someone had told me during my first few years post-TBI. The words "years post-TBI" are important for a couple of reasons. The word "years" is important because it places a realistic time frame for growth. The words post-TBI are important because I don't like the word recovery. The word recovery is a palliative that obscures the true nature of a brain injury. You are not who you were so there is nothing to recover. You are a different person after a brain injury and trying to be who you were is like trying to be someone you're not and that is a prescription for depression. To thine own self be true.

Being a new person means that who you were is gone. This is called a loss of sense of self. Overcoming this loss is hard enough, but to enjoy the fruits of growth post-TBI you must discard your second identity. This is your "TBI survivor" identity. The most difficult part of this is the *voluntary aspect*. You have to decide that you want to be more than just a victim of brain trauma.

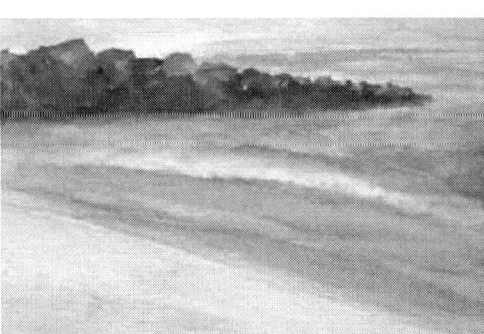

Let's be realistic, it is a very hard thing to see past

Mike Strand

your brain injury. No one can see it and you can see little else. This is, in my opinion, one of the primary reasons for support groups. Being among others who can understand your loss helps to validate your feelings and this allows you to move on and heal.

Moving beyond my brain injury and continuing to grow and develop as a person is the passion that fills my day. I am not ashamed of my brain injury, I am proud of how far I've come. I don't advertise my brain injury, but I don't hide it either. When you are ready to start your life anew I hope the following articles can help.

Sense of Self and Sense of Accomplishment

What is this "sense of self" that everyone is talking about? Your sense of self is that knowledge of what kind of person you are, how you feel and act, how you have developed over time, the roles you fill and the roles you play.

Your sense of self was turned off like a light bulb when you had your accident, when the light was turned back on the room had changed. It had become a shambles. It takes a long time to put it in order and it will never look the same. Who you are is a dynamic process. This sense, the personal experiences, are the sum of events over time. *Permit yourself the time to become a whole new person.*

How many times have you heard the phrase, "if I could do it all over again..." Well, now you can.

Brain injury is an opportunity to design yourself all over again. When you do something or behave in a way that is unsatisfactory you can tell yourself, "that wasn't me, I'm better than that." Saying it makes it so.

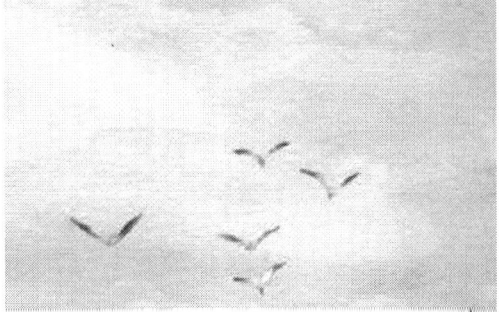

One thing that makes for a positive sense of self is a sense of accomplishment. Unlike many people, I get a real sense of accomplishment just from tying my shoes. Twelve years ago I had to learn how to do that. It was a lot of work, I still must work at it, but I'm getting better all the time. Now I only look back to see how far I've come!

Mike Strand

Post-TBI everything is hard, so it makes little difference what I'm trying to do, whether it's tying my shoes or learning another language. *I hone my will on adversity.* I started small and worked my way up. The nice thing about having no short-term memory is that it rarely occurs to me how long I've been working at something. I just put it into my routine and work at it every day until I succeed.

I believe you will find that success suits you.

Meditations

Sense of Memory

There is an oft repeated axiom, "Every brain injury is different every brain injury is the same." This is because if two people with TBI's start comparing notes they will find as many symptoms the same as different. One symptom that seems universal is loss of memory.

Even the kinds of memory lost are different. There are different degrees of long- term memory loss: some don't remember certain places or events, and some don't remember people or faces. There is also short-term memory loss, the kinds of things that you can often compensate for by writing notes and so forth. Sometimes it is not always practical to write a note, or possible to anticipate everything you will need to write down, or even if you will remember to look at your notes. However, I still find my self more likely to recall something if I have made a note than most ordinary people who try to "wing it" with just memory alone.

But what about recovering your ability to remember? So much of life's enjoyment is dependent on memory. The rich tapestry of life is etched in our memories, things such as movies, books, jokes, good times, and lessons learned.

I believe that people can improve their memory. The brain responds to activity just like a muscle. Most of us accepted having to go to physical therapy after our accidents. Many see brain injury as something different and they wait for things to just improve, or they tell themselves that they have a TBI and their memory is just bad – end of story. I refused to accept that. I worked on improving my memory and my memory has improved.

I have friends who were theater students in school. I asked them how they could memorize entire plays and they told me that it just takes practice. They also could not

Mike Strand

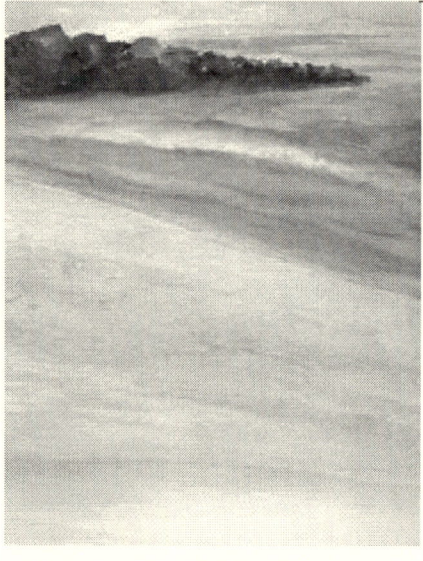

memorize as well when they started, but they found it got easier with practice. Now they just know they can do it and it is relatively easy for them.

One of the biggest oceans to cross is confidence. If you tell yourself you won't remember, or believe that you won't remember, then "voila!" you won't remember. To overcome this you need to build your confidence. Start small, try memorizing a short quote, maybe just a couple words, and work your way up from there. You are not competing with anyone. The more successes you have the stronger your confidence will become.

If you have seen the movie "Pulp Fiction" you may remember that at several times during the movie Samuel Jackson repeats the verse Ezekiel 25:17. Last year I decided I would memorize that and repeat it just the way he did in the show. It took me quite a while, I had it posted in my work area and looked at it all day long and I would listen to it on my computer at home. Now when I repeat it people just laugh and say that I must be over my brain injury if I can remember all that. I smile and tell them that I can do it in spite of my brain injury.

That last point is critical. A few years ago when I was still trying to get everyone to acknowledge my brain injury, a comment like that would have stung, as if they were denying what I went through. Now that I have made TBI a part of me instead of all of me I find it amusing, not hurtful.

One final note. Being able to memorize movie lines might be a neat parlor trick, but it has a much more important benefit. As my ability to memorize things improves, my ability to remember things improves. One quick example is I

Meditations

rarely forget to turn my headlights off when I park my car the way I always used to; this alone has already saved me money and time. I can say that I have now improved my memory to a point that it allows me a higher quality of life. Give yourself time and keep at it. The thing you should never give up on is perseverance.

Mike Strand

Sense of Compassion

One of the greatest gifts that I have realized with my brain injury is a deep sense of compassion. I have felt pain and loss very deeply and it has improved my character immensely.

Anger is a common reaction to TBI, but once you have accepted your injury and are ready to move on, that is where real growth and real compassion begin. This point may take months or years to reach, but once you are there you will find that the benefits will enrich you. Getting past that anger is beyond the scope of this article, but knowing the benefits may give you the added strength to transcend the anger.

A compassionate person is a loving person and a loving person is a loved person. Everyone wants to be loved. TBI gives us a bridge to compassion.

People are not drawn to you by your needs; if anything, a needy person pushes them away. We are drawn to people by their compassion. You must be strong for someone else before they will be strong for you. When you are strong for someone you will find it makes you stronger, regardless of what they do or don't do. It is like a confidence building exercise.

So many brain-injured people are lonely and that is unfortunate. It is doubly unfortunate because they have been given a gift that empowers them to draw others to them. When you develop that inner calm and strength that comes from mastering a difficult situation like TBI, you will draw others to you.

Sympathy says, "I know how you feel."
Empathy says, "How can I help?"
Volunteering is one way to demonstrate compassion.

Meditations

Anyone who has heard Craig Martinson, a survivor from Minnesota, speak about volunteering knows the rewards that such compassion has to offer.

Compassion involves you immediately with others. Thus, you cannot act compassionately and be alone at the same time. People will see your compassion even if it's not directed at them and be drawn towards you. As the Hindus say, "The breath of the compassionate is never taken alone."

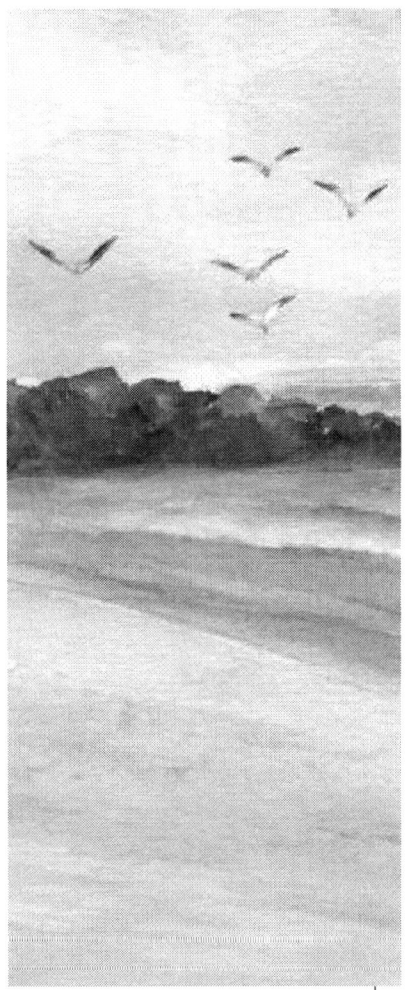

Mike Strand

A Tip for Faster Recovery

So many times when we ask what we can do to get better we are told to be patient, it just takes time. Attitude is the most important in my opinion, but that's not really doing anything. So what can one do?

Well, I came across something the other day, which I believe is just what many people are looking for. This is a study that shows a definite improvement in mental faculties. This study was done on older people and was connected to age-related brain issues, but I think survivors will find this relevant.

A study was done by Professor Arthur Kramer on what the effects of simply walking regularly would have on mental functions. Specifically, the study focused on reversing the aging process, which is very similar to brain injury recovery. What he found out will not surprise very many people: exercise is good for you. *What* will raise many eyebrows is *how* good it is for you. One-half his test subjects walked for half an hour three times a week, and the other half remained sedentary (inactive). The active people improved up to 15% on mental tests!

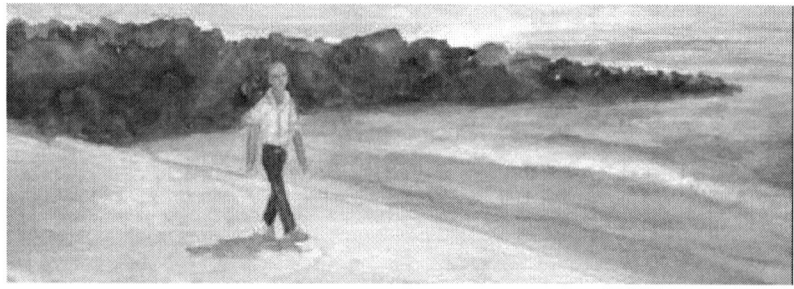

Meditations

The areas most improved were regions responsible for "executive control functions." Those are the areas with which, as brain injured people, we suffer some of our most debilitating deficits. You know the issues I'm talking about—planning, and using working memory, making decisions, and picking out relevant information from irrelevant distractions.

These tests were conducted on elderly people, so even older TBI sufferers can expect some benefit from exercise, and one would imagine that younger folks might even expect more dramatic results.

Of course, it is always a good idea to consult with your doctor before embarking on any exercise program. Also, you should try to find something that you enjoy doing so that you are more likely to keep doing it. Good luck!

Mike Strand

Act Happy to Be Happy

Depression is almost certain with TBI. In fact, I would say that if you suffer a traumatic brain injury and don't get depressed, then you just don't get it. I did not become clinically depressed until about two years after my accident. It took until then for the double vision, the dizziness, the confusion, and the fact that I never felt good, to finally overwhelm me. Like many people, I despised the idea of being dependent on any medication and the thought of what those drugs would be doing to the rest of my body was just as disturbing. However, when depression finally ran through me, I surrendered to my doctor's advice and went on antidepressant medication. I adhered strictly to the prescribed regimen so as to affect the greatest efficacy and speediest recovery. Ultimately, this took almost a year.

I was determined to do everything that I could to avoid becoming depressed in the future. I have determined two ways that have kept me free of depression ever since. The first way is one that I believe will work for everyone. The second way is a path that is different for each person and I only relate mine as an example.

About eight years ago I went to a seminar given by a doctor who had studied the effects of smiling and laughter on the health of the individual. We all know that depression is a chemical imbalance. Long after the original cause of the depression may be gone the imbalance remains and this is what we call clinical depression. We know that when somebody is depressed they look depressed, their posture is bad, their shoulders droop, their head sinks, they don't smile, and so forth. According to medical research, it is this physical state that induces the body to manufacture the chemical imbalance that makes one unhappy. This chemical change must be

Meditations

overcome to be happy again. But how? "Simple," said the good doctor, "just smile." If you change your face from a frown to a smile, if you sit up straight, your body will eventually change its chemistry. Look at yourself in the mirror with a big grin on your face—how could you stay unhappy? The dissonance is startling. You have the power to smile. If you are able to get over yourself and let the smile work its magic, you will find your mood improving. I can't suggest you do this as a way of treating severe depression, but it can't hurt. I believe quite strongly that it has helped me.

Laughter is even stronger than smiling. We have all heard the adage that "laughter is the best medicine." Well, it didn't come out of nothingness. Laughter is the strongest prescription available for pain and depression. It releases endorphins from the body's own pharmacy. Have you ever been carrying something heavy and started laughing at something funny? Laughing so hard you had to set down what you were carrying for fear of dropping it? That's endorphins numbing your pain and relaxing those muscles. Watching a funny movie or joking around with friends is some of the most effective therapy I know of for treating pain or low spirits.

The second method is spirituality. Almost without exception, I have found that most survivors have a deep and abiding faith that sustains them. As an atheist, this didn't really work for me. I know there are others out there that also share my lack of faith, and although my spirituality is very private, I would like to share the path that I have followed to happiness. I have turned to Buddhism, I am not a Buddhist per se, but I have found strength in the teachings of the Dalai Lama. There is a mystical side to Bhuddism that I do not embrace, but the teachings are very relevant. The book

Mike Strand

I recommend is called *The Art of Happiness* by the Dalai Lama and Howard C. Cutler, M.D. This book combines the teachings of the Dalai Lama with the interpretation of a psychologist.

These two techniques have been the cornerstone of my recovery that has allowed me to face the challenges and the heartbreaks of brain injury recovery.

Meditations

Beyond Language

Communicating with language is very difficult with most people that suffer from TBI. We have the idea in our mind, we may even have the sentence on the tip of our tongue, but it just doesn't come out as we mean it to. As a demonic corollary, the more passionately we feel about something, the less it is likely that we are going to be able to say what we mean.

The way we try to compensate for this is by taking repeated stabs at it. We try stating again and again in different ways what we are trying to say, all the while feeliing as though we are losing our audience until we can't even remember what we were trying to say. AAAARRRGH!

You would think that we would learn. Better to remain silent and be thought a fool than to open our mouths and remove all doubt. A big part of communication is effectively sharing your anger and frustration and that is not something I have mastered or even feel confident I can explore in an article like this. That is why there are people with degrees making a lot of money dealing with those issues.

What I would like to talk about is communicating positively with friends and loved ones, and being the kind of communicator that draws people towards you instead of pushing them away.

We all want someone to talk to. We all want someone who will hear our problems. We do not need someone to solve our problems. We especially don't need pop-psychologists and their breezy replies like "you just gotta do what makes you happy." We just want someone who will listen.

There is our solution. Just listen. If people know you as someone who is a good listener they will seek you out.

Mike Strand

This is an ideal situation for us because it doesn't matter what you say, what matters is what you don't say. All you have to say is what they just told you. For example:

    Them: "I am really teed off today."
    You: "You're really teed off?"
    Them: "My mom is driving me up a wall."
    You: "Why is your mom driving you up a wall?"
    Them: "Well, today she..."

You get the point I'm sure. Just practice this a little bit and you will be surprised at how people respond. They will find they like spending time with you.

When it comes to the "international language," the language of love, we should find ourselves even better off. You will have to make a conscious effort, however. You know how when a person is blind their other senses become heightened in order to compensate? The same can be true for verbal communication. All you need to do is watch an old silent movie and you will see that they were able to convey all the drama and pathos without words, maybe even more so than movies with words. If you are in a romantic relationship, I suggest that you try an evening without words. It will be difficult at first, but it gets easier. If someone gets angry, start talking! The point of this game is greater communication, if someone gets angry and turns off, then you have stopped communicating and that is the opposite of what you are trying to accomplish.

If you only take one point from this article, let it be this: When it comes to verbal communication and brain injury, less is more.

Meditations

Boredom

My friend Carlos had a period during his adolescence when he didn't have much to do. You know that age, too old for all the stuff you used to do, but not old enough to do all the things you wanted to do. Well, he came across a whole pile of rubber bands, an almost limitless supply. So he rolled one into a little ball and then he grabbed another one and wrapped it around the first one. That was so much fun and so rewarding that he selected one more rubber band and repeated the process. He did this whenever he had some spare time and wasn't going anywhere for awhile. By the end of the summer he had a rubber band ball about the size of a basketball. He called his creation "Boredom." Boredom became an institution to us. We took it wherever we went. That was twenty years ago. The last place I remember boredom was at college, in the Student Governing Board offices, where it was our constant companion.

Even before I had left the hospital, boredom had found me again. In my opinion, the hardest thing about brain injury is the boredom. Everyone finds being infirm to be boring, but brain injury lasts forever! If not forever, for an uncomfortably long time. Everyone with brain injury has memory problems, but everyone can still remember how much fun they used to have and how interesting their life was before their brain injury.

It's like the football player who is injured and told he will never play football again, except you were playing life and now it appears you will never play life again. What do you tell those well-meaning people who want to give you a kind word of support when they ask what's wrong? Do you look at them straight on and say, "I'm bored." In the work-a-day world where people are longing for some peace and quiet, how do you convey the utter futility of your predicament? It's like you're waiting to get better, but that's years away, if even then.

I do remember the first year after my accident, not in detail, but in general. I remember how bored I was. I still get bored, I think I will spend my life running from boredom. The difference between now and then is that now I'm not bored all the time. I have discovered a secret. The opposite of boredom is purpose. If you find a purpose to your life you will have a way to alleviate boredom. Purpose fills each day with opportunity and each moment with wonder. I actually find myself lamenting that there aren't enough hours in the day!

The tough part is actually finding a purpose. In my experience it is rarely found by sitting back and wondering what it might be, wishing upon a star. Usually, people are going through their life and this purpose just bites them on the nose. This isn't much solace for those who are bored now, so what can a person do?

I would look at volunteer opportunities. This is not to say that this is the best way to find your passion and purpose in life, but it does give you something to do until you find your place in the world.

Remember to look inward. Before I was of much use to anyone, I spent time improving myself. "Invest in yourself first," a sage once told me. That is my mantra now. Whenever I talk about brain injury to survivors I talk about ways that I found to improve myself after my accident, using many of these techniques I have written about in these pages, but everyone is different and we all must chart our own course.

Good luck and happy sailing.

Giving Yourself Credit

One of the most common complaints about brain injury is that no one can "see" your disability. We look fine and even among people who know we are brain injured we often find our disability is overlooked. Add to that the fact that so many have no idea what a brain injury is all about, and you've got a recipe for misunderstanding and alienation. This is one of the many reasons we are impatient for our complete recovery.

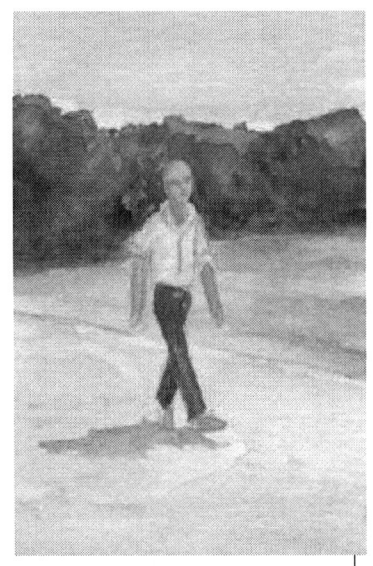

One of the most common complaints heard in any support group is frustration over the length of recovery. There is so much pain and so much hard work and so little reward. Day after day we face the same dull tasks, day after day we don't seem to get better, and if we do improve they just raise the bar and we start over from square one. Its like being in training for the Olympics except that there is no gold medal, no adoring crowd, and no cheesy interviews from network personas in cheap suits.

There are many aspects to the outside world that we cannot change. Recovery is slow and difficult, but we can change our perspective.

That is what I decided to do. I was as bad as all the other people who would look at me and see no brain injury,

Mike Strand

who would see nothing amiss. I had to reevaluate my position; I was in such bad shape after my accident that I almost died. What I needed was a big gash or bruise on my head to remind my self that I was horribly injured, some sort of mark that could visually remind me just how hurt I was. Since that was not to be, I just had to consider how far I had come. I had to realize just what a complicated piece of machinery the brain is. Skin can just scar over and the wound is healed. The brain doesn't use scars. Scars are the body's duct tape, tie wire, and Bondo, that can cover up a damaged chassis. Repairing a high performance engine will use none of those things and is a much a more involved and delicate process. If an engine is damaged severely enough, it may never run as well as it used to—I accept that. It was time to accept that my brain may never run as well as it used to.

Fortunately my heart can compensate for my brain. I believe this has made me a better person than I ever was before. As difficult as it is sometimes, I have to ignore what I've lost and focus on what I have gained. Now, the only reason I look back is to see how far I've come.

Meditations

On Being Well Liked

One thing we all need, not just TBI survivors, but everyone, is for people to like us. How come some people have lots of friends and others don't. I will tell you what works for me. Many people will say, "Well of course you have lots of friends, Mike. You're so good looking and funny and smart, but what about everyone else?" Actually, I'm joking, nobody says that about me. So just why do I have so many friends?

I have many friends because I like people. I'm not shy about it either. When I meet someone I am genuinely pleased to have made his or her acquaintance. When somebody I know walks in the room I am glad to see them, as if I was alone in the room until they showed up.

In conversation, I try to talk about something I know they are interested in. If I don't know what they are interested in I will try to notice what they are wearing and tell them I like it.

The single most likeable thing about someone is how much he or she likes you. The important thing to note about that is that it gives you a lot of control over how others feel about you. The trick is to give others the benefit of the doubt. Assume that you have met your new best friend when you are introduced to someone. If you find out otherwise later you can just move on, no harm done.

One piece of advice: avoid talking about yourself. Unless you are asked a question, talk about them. If you don't know enough to talk about them then ask about them. If they ask about you, be polite and answer briefly. Save full disclosures for another time. If you want people to see past your brain injury, then you have to see past your brain injury. Here's an example:

Mike Strand

Them: So you have a brain injury?
You: Yes.
Them: So how did it happen, if you don't mind me asking?
You: No, I don't mind. I was in a motor vehicle accident.
Them: Are you all better now?
You: Actually, I still have quite a few problems.
Them: I bet its tough. I have a brother-in-law who fell off a platform at work...
You: How is he doing?

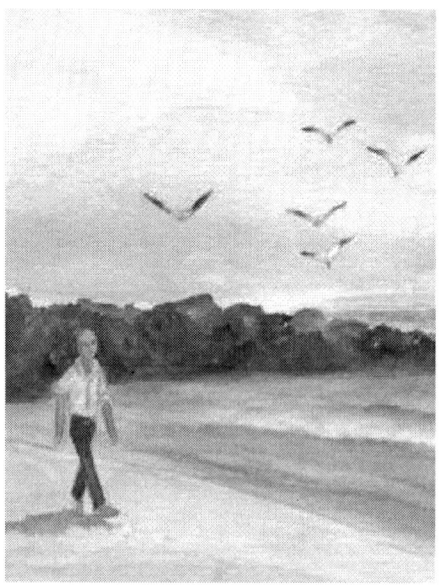

It's usually the case that someone knows someone with a brain injury. Show concern for THAT person—are they getting the help they need? Have they contacted the Brain Injury Association? When people ask about your injury they are usually just being polite; be polite and respond briefly. When you ask about someone they mention, you are just being polite, after all. This is how civil society works.

Good friendships with quality people take time and constant effort. If you wish to attract and keep quality people, then you have to work at being a quality person yourself.

Meditations

Learning to See

I see the world differently now. I see it with "TBI Vision." I'm not talking about my double vision, or the difficulty my brain has in processing the information my eyes are taking in. Those are very real and serious limitations. What I am talking about is the *way* I see things now.

All too often, ordinary people get caught up in what they see. They place too much emphasis on what is plainly right before their eyes. If something doesn't square with the facts then it must not be so. "A is A" as Aristotle said. "Ding an Sich" (a thing in itself) as Kant said. Time and again it is repeated that we gain knowledge of our world through direct observation. None of these beliefs allow for brain injury, where that information is confused, obfuscated, or just plain missed.

This would seem to imply that a brain-injured person is less able to operate effectively in the world. In many cases this is just not so. Blind people can operate effectively, as we know. In fact, many blind people who get their sight are unhappy with what they see; the "real world" is not a world they are comfortable in.

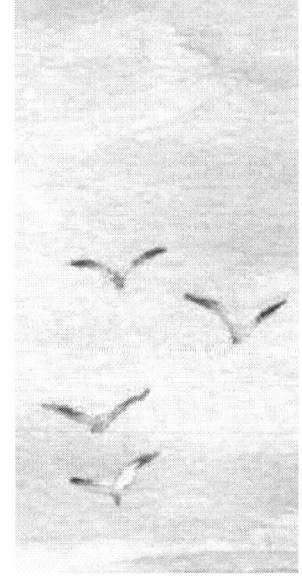

This is an insight into what I mean when I say that I am glad for my TBI and would not wish it away even if I could. I see so much more with my heart and I would not want to give that up. I use to see the world in very cold and hostile terms. Now I see it in warmer friendlier terms. Has the world changed? No, I have. Instead of only seeing what is, I also see what can be.

It was a long and arduous process to come to this knowing. Now that I have it I would not give it up. This is what I mean when I say that I am glad to have sustained a severe TBI. All the pressure is off. No one expects me to be the best, or the smartest, or the richest. All I have to do is be the best me I can be. I can be a good friend, a good volunteer, and a valued person.

I live my life with passion. I care. I laugh. I love. All of these are things that I gain by sharing them; they make me a wealthy soul. Because I want these things in my life (and who does not?), I give them away. They rebound back to me. I like myself when I am this way, and when I like myself I find others like me also. I ask no one for compassion, joy, or love. I simply give it unconditionally and I find my own cup overflowing.

This is how I choose to see the world; this is my "TBI vision."

Meditations

A Memory Like All Others

What do you think these three people have in common?

1. A man tees up a golf ball and hits it straight down the fairway. After waiting a few moments for his partner to hit, the man tees up his ball again, forgetting that he hit the first drive.
2. A man puts his glasses down on the edge of a couch. Several minutes later he realizes that he can't find the glasses, and spends half an hour searching his home before locating them.
3. A man temporarily places a violin on the top of his car. Forgetting that he has done so, he drives off with the violin still perched on the top of the roof.

If you guessed that they are all men you have guessed correctly, but that is not my point. What else do they all have in common?

None of these people have a brain injury.

I have recently completed reading a book by Daniel L. Schacter, the chair of Harvard University's Department of Psychology, titled *The Seven Sins of Memory : How the Mind Forgets and Remembers*. In this book he outlines seven different ways the mind manages to forget. Seven different ways!

Of course, he makes many valid points and observations, but I was looking at more than just his observations and conclusions. I was trying to determine if there would be anything valuable for a brain injured person to learn from such a book.

After reading the dozens of accounts of people's mnemonic shortcomings in the book, I was able to make one salient observation. Everyone has an imperfect memory; our memory may be more imperfect than most, but ordinary people are constantly hampered by memory failure.

Mike Strand

I'm not going to say that we have nothing to complain about, because if it's bad for other people, it is that much worse for us. What I am going to suggest is that there are definite ways we can work to improve our memories. If other people can do it, so can we. Our hurdles may be higher, and the road fraught with increased perils...So what else is new?

As always, the first step is attitude. In *Illusions,* Richard Bach says, "argue for your limitations, and sure enough, they're yours." The mind is surprisingly obedient; if we tell ourselves we can't do something then we can't. If you first say that you can't, you're almost never wrong.

Unfortunately, the corollary is not true. If you believe you can do something, it doesn't necessarily mean you can. I'm just saying, as a first step, you must believe you can succeed.

Tatiana Cooley, the 1999 National Memory Champion can remember thousands of numbers in a series as well as other memory feats. What she cannot do is get through a day without post-it notes and a day planner. She is terribly absent-minded. The reasons for this are explained in Dr. Schacter's book, but basically, there are two different kinds of memory at work here and one she is able to improve on and the other she sacrifices.

Imagine an ordinary person forgetting something—they probably will quickly dismiss it as just another memory failure in a long list of mnemonic shortcomings. If you or I forget something, we say, "it's my brain injury."

The only people I have ever heard of who have had excellent memories are people who subsequently sustained a brain injury. Apparently, the best way to guard against a TBI is to have a bad memory to start with. I'm being facetious here, but I am making a point. We often remember our memory as being much better than it was. The logic of the last sentence is clear. Dr. Schacter calls this the sin of bias. This is what is normally called seeing the past through rose colored glasses. It is a natural condition of memory. Not surprisingly, it is that much more pronounced in a TBI survivor. We need to be easier on ourselves.

In summary, let me say this: Our memories are worse than most people's memories. Everyone has to use

Meditations

various compensatory strategies to make it through a day and it is more so for us. There are strategies to improve memory, though we have to realize that it is going to be harder for us, and we will accomplish less. Maybe this all seems dark and foreboding; the light to draw from what I am saying is that there is hope. Set realistic goals and expect to work hard, when you succeed you will be that much more rewarded. As Thomas Paine said, "What we obtain too cheap, we esteem to lightly."

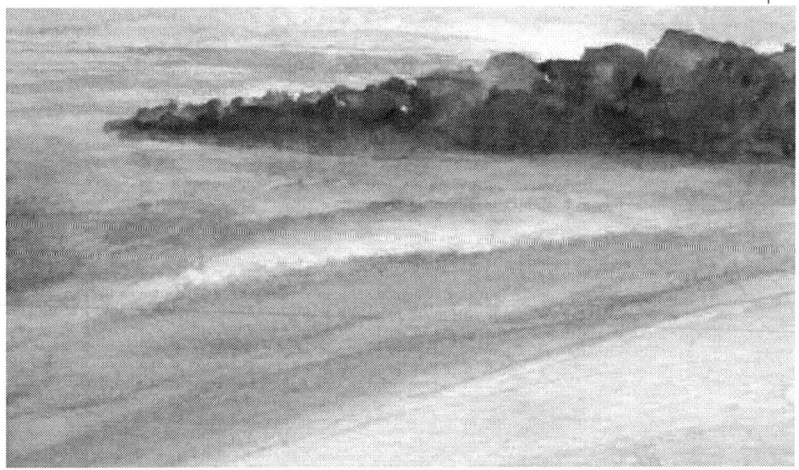

Mike Strand

Meta-cognition: Thinking about Thinking

Recent studies have overturned the long held belief that as you get older your brain gets weaker and more inefficient. The brain does not get worse with age; bad habits erode the mind. New brain cells are constantly being grown in the hippocampus and the brain is always building new pathways.

The brain is like a muscle. With use it will grow stronger. With disuse it will atrophy. Unlike many other organs of the body, it never wears out, but it does fade out from lack of stimulus.

Many people find themselves trapped after brain injury—trapped in a body with a brain that cannot do what it used to. So they sit and wait to get better. Unfortunately, that's not how brain injury recovery works. Brain injury recovery *is* work. The work doesn't have to be unpleasant, but it must be fairly consistent. It is only by dogged determination that limitations can be overcome.

A word about limitations: limitations aren't permanent. Limitations are markers that say how far you've gone in the past. They say nothing about the future except how much further you have left to go. View your limitations as the highest rung you've ever reached on a ladder. You can always try to go one rung higher.

At any point in your recovery you may not get any better. The doctors really can't give the families or the victims of brain injury any definite answers to the questions, "How long till I get better?" and "Will I regain this or that ability?" They cannot wave a magic wand or give you a magic drug that will make you whole again

Take control of your brain's functions. Accept that your brain is an amazing organ and that you can make it

Meditations

better and stronger. How good and how strong is up to you. You can always improve, but there may be a point of diminishing returns. You must decide how you want to proceed.

Your brain can be very obedient. It will do what you ask of it. Program your brain to perform a certain task within a certain time limit. Tell yourself that you will complete a task within a certain (reasonable) time. You will be surprised at how much more you can accomplish. They have tested for this under laboratory conditions and it is a fact that if you give yourself a goal and a time limit the brain tends to work faster and more successfully.

Acknowledge your limitations and devise techniques for working around them. Instead of saying "I can't remember," try saying "I will remember when X happens." Give yourself a command such as, "When I park my car I will shut my lights off." Visualize doing this. When my wife asks me to pick up certain items for her when I go shopping I visualize selecting the item when I get to that part of the store. This works for me provided she doesn't ask for too many things and that I know where the item is so I can visualize it. With practice you can actually get quite proficient at this sort of thing. As always, start with baby steps. Success builds success.

Visualization is a key that you can use to improve your brainpower. It is a tool that you can use to fight the failure mechanism that we all struggle with. When we tell ourselves, "I must remember," it is usually with this nagging feeling that we will forget. When you visualize actually remembering to do something, you override that failure impulse.

So, you start by taking control of your brain's functions. Your brain is very obedient and will respond to commands. This does take practice. Practice being successful at something. Acknowledge your limitations. Visualize yourself being successful.

I am not talking about saving a drowning child, landing a crippled airplane, or curing a wasting disease. I'm talking about wearing matching socks, turning off the stove, and calling your mother on her birthday. We can be successful people.

Meditations

On Being Dependent

One of the most difficult things about brain injury for me was the helplessness. I was not used to being taken care of. I was used to being independent and strong and letting others lean on me. After my accident it was always a constant battle, striving to recover and yet yielding to assistance when necessary. It was a balancing act and it was one I wasn't very good at.

Facilitating a support group gave me a whole new perspective. It allowed me to view my situation through the eyes of others. Listening to caregivers and victims sharing their feelings I was able to be on the outside looking in. For the first time I was able to imagine how my wife must feel and I was able to hear how I must sound to her. This new knowledge is one of the rewards that I have found in being a facilitator. My only regret is that it took me ten years to figure this out.

A brain injury is tough and it is overwhelming. One of the first things I was faced with was that many of the things that brought me joy were now beyond my reach. It was often easy to feel like there was nothing left to live for. I saw all my dreams shattered. I felt I had been cheated and I had lived my life to completion. As I often do in dark moments of despair I turned to *Illusions* by Richard Bach, my favorite book. I paged through it looking for an answer and this is what I found:

Here is a test to see if your mission in life is over.
    If you're alive,
                it isn't.

Mike Strand

I'm just one person, but in my ten years post-TBI I keep finding reasons to be here. Open your heart and touch a life; there is never a shortage of those who need someone to lend an ear.

At times I honestly felt there was nothing left to live for, but in saying so I was telling others that they are not worth living for. I can now imagine how that must have hurt. They were helping me because they loved me, not because they pitied me, which is the way I felt. I decided I must never esteem the love of others too lightly!

I had always been the strong one. The one all others could lean on and draw from my seemingly inexhaustible reservoir of strength. Now it was time to accept that I had to be taken care of, and that I must yield the care giving responsibilities to others, especially those I had previously taken care of. The shoe was on the other foot! So, as much as I may not have liked this new arrangement, all the wishing in the world wouldn't make it otherwise. I had to face reality.

This didn't mean I would stop trying. If anything, the way I feel should motivate me to do whatever is required to expedite my recovery. Until then I can accept help. All false independence does is make everyone miserable. The least I can do is be thankful, humble, and cherish the love I receive from others.

This is how I have decided to view my world. This should make my path a little easier to traverse and I know it will make the lives of my caregivers more rewarding. We live for them as they live for us.

Meditations

Real Healing

A reporter asked me recently, "How long did your recovery take?" My stock reply was that you never fully recover from brain injury, that most people see the lion's share of recovery within the first two years. All of that is factual, but none of it is correct.

It is like asking, "How long does it take to grow up?" Growing up is a process that never really ends. One does tend to develop in different ways as one gets older and at some point we consider ourselves "grown up." However, you never really stop growing.

The same is true for brain injury. There can be discrete measurable gains after brain injury that can be described as recovery, but beyond that there is the intangible of personal growth.

Part of this personal growth I like to label healing. Healing is the act of reconstructing ourselves after the "loss of self" that is part of brain injury.

The first step is to accept that we have a brain injury. This is more than just acknowledging the fact that it happened. It is accepting the fact that you are not the person you were. Trying to be the person you were is living in the past. When you are truly ready to be who you are, you are ready to move on.

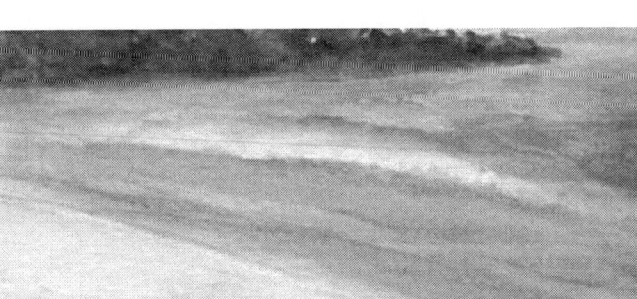

Mike Strand

The second step is to get over it. It is all too easy to try and hold on to the deficits of brain injury. It becomes so very much a part of who you are, that to move beyond it is like losing yourself all over again. Yes you have deficits, but you are you in spite of your deficits, and THAT is what makes you a better person.

The third step is to find value in the experience. It is restitution for the soul. Restitution is the act of putting right what is wrong. This is the true nature of healing. If you do not see your brain injury as valuable, then your brain injury has accomplished nothing. This is completely your choice. I found that my brain injury knocked me off my high horse and allowed me to become a more compassionate person. Compassion has unlocked riches I would have never received. My world is now larger and encompasses broader horizons than I would have ever imagined. We must all find that which has value to us. This will be different for everyone and is part of this fortune hunt called life that is far too fleeting.

Meditations

A Routine Gift

Routine is a constant reference as to when and where I am. With brain injury one realizes just how fragile our awareness of place and time really is. I can be at the mall with my wife and be looking at something while she walks away. I will look up and suddenly nothing is as I suspected and I will feel this sudden panic as I try to reorient myself, try to find some clue that will tell me where I am and when I am. Not just what time it is, or just what day it is, but what year is it? How old am I? A split second of panic until I regain my perspective.

Routine allows me to compensate for my lack of initiative. I may not notice that the house needs vacuuming, but I know that on Mondays I vacuum. It is good to make lists for many things, but inserting something into my routine allows me to do a number of tasks that would overwhelm me if I saw them all on a list. Routine allows me to be a more effective person.

Most people view routine as boring. "Boring as compared to what?" I ask. "Boring as compared to being confused and inactive?" I query. Variety is very important. Many people are distracted from accomplishing long-term goals because they want immediate variety. I get my variety long-term because routine keeps the distractions at bay. Day by day my routine may seem boring, but I've accomplished so very much in the last eleven years since my brain injury! *These are things I would never have even considered doing before.* In addition to doing all the tasks you might imagine in an ordinary life (I prefer "ordinary" to "normal"), I also run five miles several times a week, I read seventy pages a day, I ran for Lt. Governor in 1994 and 1998, I expect to get the Libertarian party's nomination for Governor in 2002, I

Mike Strand

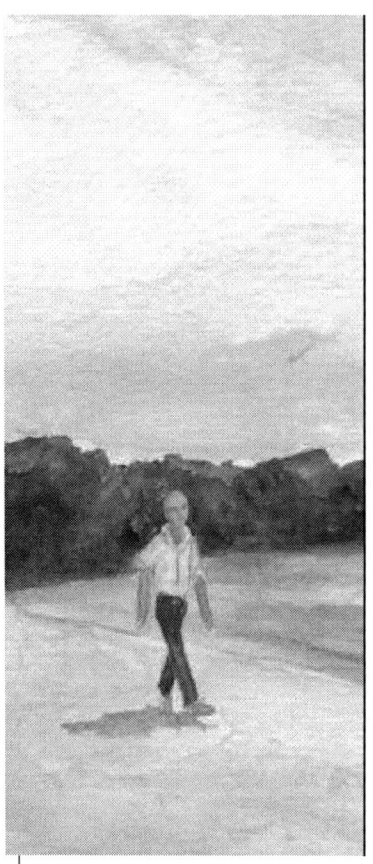

facilitate the Stillwater support group, I speak four languages besides English, and my writing has appeared in a few Libertarian publications as well as in the brain injury newsletter, I designed and built a teaching aid to show the effects of time distortion at relative speeds, I protested the stadium tax increase, and more.

I don't list all that to brag. I'm certainly no genius and I sure don't have limitless energy. It just really amazes me how much a person can do if you just put it into a routine and doggedly persist. I don't question whether or not I want to do something on a daily basis, I just get up and do it. I face each day with child-like wonder and boundless curiosity. Oh yes, and as always, I hone my will on adversity.

Self-image and Brain Injury

Self-image is a big concern for survivors. So much of what we think of ourselves is bound up in who we were, not who we are. We hear again and again that we have to let go of our old selves and embrace our new selves. Well those are great words, but it isn't that easy.

It is not easy to embrace this new you when this new you is but a shade of who you were in so many ways. It is impossible to overlook the way you were and they way you are and not feel a sense of loss and regret. You compare the pictures before and after and it is difficult not to feel inadequate.

The only way I know to do deal with this is to counter the poor self-image. I have found a way that works for me. I do things that make me feel good about myself. So much of the time we focus on doing what makes us feel good. This does not last. If we focus on doing things that make us feel good about ourselves, this lasts. I feel good about myself when I show compassion for another. This is something that anyone can do. In spite of that, we never seem to have enough compassion in the world.

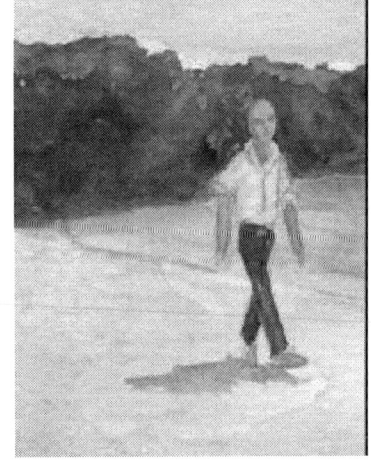

Let me restate. Do things that make you feel good about yourself. I like this strategy because it puts me in control. We all want to feel like we have more control in our lives and this is pro-active.

Mike Strand

There is another benefit to compassion. It is a good way to get your mind off your problems. Don't worry about your problems. I find that even if I think about something else, or someone else, I can usually get in touch with all my problems at my earliest convenience. If I have forgotten about a problem I can probably get along just fine without it anyway.

Seriously, one of the best ways to deal with your problems is to immerse yourself in helping others. It is almost impossible to feel powerless over your situation when you are helping another. Giving is a supremely selfish act. It makes you feel very good. If it did not you would not be doing it. Gain strength through enlightened self-interest.

Soul Gazing

Words are one way to communicate with others. They are not the only way, and for many survivors they are a difficult and frustrating way to share information. Of course, for most situations the spoken word is the best way we have to converse.

After TBI, it is often times very difficult to maintain a romantic relationship. Communication issues are some of the biggest reasons relationships fail and for those suffering from or with a TBI, it is even more so.

A brain injury can change a romantic relationship on many levels. First and foremost, the person is probably a whole different individual, roles may have changed dramatically, the spouse of a brain-injured person may feel like they have lost a mate and gained a child.

I think it is important to reconnect on a very intimate level. Intimacy is the single aspect most unique to a romantic relationship. There is a technique that may help. It is called "soul gazing."

To practice soul gazing you simply sit opposite one another. Each person focuses on their partner's left eye with both of their eyes. The eyes truly are the windows of the soul. Soul gazing is completely non-verbal, although you may play soft instrumental music and light a candle. You also want to minimize distractions. Along with minimizing distractions, you should also refrain from any other contact such as holding hands. To maximize the effect you should concentrate on the eyes. You can experiment with how far apart your faces are during the exercise. Start a couple feet away and gradually move closer until you are almost kissing. For an even greater intimacy you can alternate your breathing so one person is inhaling while the other is exhaling, sharing breath like this is the ultimate in bonding.

Mike Strand

How long you do this for is dependent on you. At first you may just do it for a minute or so. Eventually, couples might extend it for quite a while.

One of the hardest things about soul gazing is not laughing. Being this intimate is very uncomfortable for many people and the normal reaction to this kind of discomfort is to laugh. If this happens, just let your self laugh and then relax and try again. Keep at it and eventually you'll get it.

That is all there is to it. This won't fix everything, but it is something you can try to make your relationship stronger. It is a way to communicate without having to speak. As is so often the case with TBI, we must think outside the box.

The Really Scary Thing About TBI

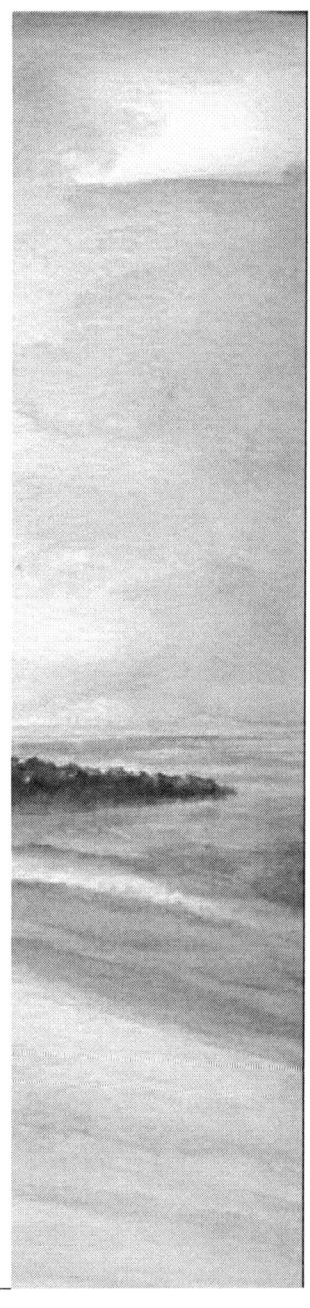

Things I can remember fall into three categories: The things I only think about doing and then think I have done, The things I dream that I did and then think that I have done, and the things I have actually done and then think that I have done. This means that to the best of my memory, when I think that I have done something, I have about a 33% chance of actually having done it.

Fortunately, more often than not I actually have done those things that I think I have done. For those of you recently injured (less than about five years,) take heart— it tends to occur more and more over time. Still, every once in a while, I think I have done something, when in fact I only thought about doing it, or dreamt that I did it. Since I rarely remember my dreams anymore, dreaming I did something is even more confusing.

If any non-TBI sufferers read those last paragraphs and find them confusing, then perhaps you have glimpsed how disconcerting the confusion surrounding a brain injury can be. You know how it is when you have a dream and it makes sense until you try and explain it to someone

Mike Strand

else? Imagine further that you can't just laugh it off and say it was only a dream. Welcome to the TBI world.

In a dream, random things can seem plausible. This is how reality often seems to a TBI survivor. People are constantly telling you that things are not as you perceive them to be. Sometimes you are right, sometimes you are not, and the difference can seem very arbitrary.

In the movie "Vanilla Sky," the audience spends most of the movie not knowing if a certain sequence is a dream or reality. This very unsettling feeling gnaws at you and you find yourself frantically watching the show and impatiently waiting for the moment when you can see the "big" picture. This is very similar to the way a TBI survivor feels every day, all the time.

It is an icky feeling. It's kind of cool in the movie, because the movie only lasts so long, and there is an end that puts it all together. Of course, with a brain injury, it never goes away and it never comes together. Eventually you become numb to it, until something happens, like you were sure you went to the mall and had that spare key made, only now you wonder if you went, and if so, where the key is. Instantly your world seems very surreal. The more you try to pinpoint reality the farther it recedes – just like the evanescent dream which seems clear in your mind until you try to remember something particular about it, and then it seems to vanish.

"What is real?" is a big question. Add to that "what *was* real?" and you get a maelstrom of possibilities that boggle the mind and you find yourself in another vertigo spiral. Welcome to the TBI world.

Meditations

The Sleeper Awakens

Everyone is capable of much more than regular life asks of him or her. This is proved when you watch the news and they talk about some accident or disaster and the "heroes" that rise up out of the rank and file of every day life to deal with the traumatic event. Rarely are these people who have any claim to fame or greatness other than they were just there and they did what had to be done.

This is not to belittle what they accomplish. In fact, it is a solemn salute to the great things that are regularly achieved by those who are faced with an overwhelming hurdle.

My brain injury was the bitterest pill I ever had to swallow. I always felt inwardly that I could handle anything that life dished out, as long as I had my mind to rely on. I somehow felt that if my mind were damaged I wouldn't want to be saved. Coincidentally, that's where I got hit, right in the mind.

Much to my surprise, even *that* didn't make me give up. A part of me that I had never had to rely on was there when I needed it. In mystical terms, this is that time when

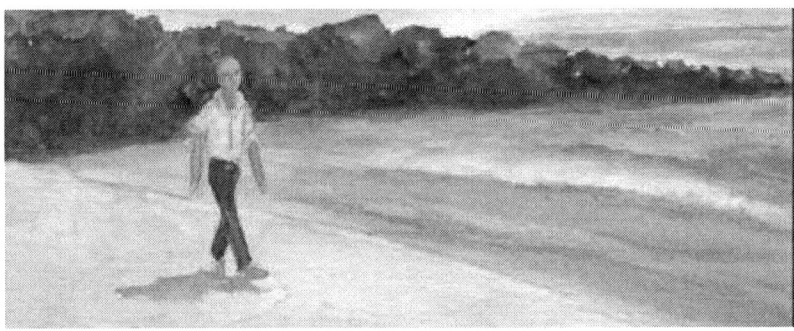

Mike Strand

"the sleeper awakens." That is the inner strength you never knew you had. This is Clark Kent diving into a phone booth and emerging as Superman to save the day. This is that part of you that, when you find yourself trembling on a rocky ledge about to fall, screams "no!" and pulls you back. This is that part of you that finds the courage to turn around and walk the razor's edge, face the fire, or just get out of bed.

Brain injury is your opportunity to be great. Most people live whole lives waiting for something to happen to them to make them great. Lucky us. We've been pre-selected for greatness. Hey, nobody said being great was easy. I am great-full. If I had anymore greatness I'd be depressed. My plate of great is overflowing. No more greatness for me thank you, I'll leave some for the next guy.

Seriously, it's all a matter of perspective. This is just one way to look at brain injury. It's important to note that you aren't great because you've had a brain injury, but you can be great because of what you do in reaction to your brain injury.

Meditations

Owning Your Brain Injury

Most of us spend some time wallowing around in denial and this is natural. It takes awhile to accept that this really happened and you are not just having a bad dream.

A sign that you've accepted your brain injury is when you first take responsibility for your injury. I'm not saying it is your fault; blame is irrelevant. Being responsible means accepting that recovery is no one else's job more than yours. You have to decide that you want to get better. You have to decide that you want it bad enough to work at it. Being willing to work at it means that you aren't going to be hung up on the end result. It means that you want recovery so bad that you are willing to work at it even though you have little or no success. There's no point in giving up because you can't go back.

I can't guarantee you'll recover successfully. I can guarantee that you will grow. It's not reaching the destination that makes you a better person; it's the journey. If we have an advantage over ordinary folks it is that we are on a

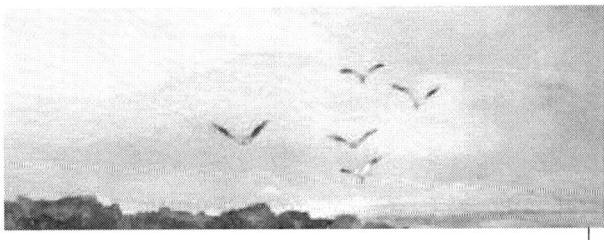

seemingly perpetual journey that's all uphill. To quote Bill Murray in the movie "Stripes," "Talk about massive potential for growth, I am the acorn that becomes the mighty oak!"

Mike Strand

Towards a Better Life

We can all work so hard on recovering from our brain injury that we forget what makes us happy. We get to thinking, if we could only get better, get back to normal (ordinary), everything would be so much better.

Eliminating the negative will not give us the positive. If we just focus on fixing what is wrong we will miss all the things that make for real happiness. Just fixing what is wrong won't make us happy, and at any rate, considering brain injury, that is not an option.

Life can be beautiful if we don't try to live in a dream world. If we try to envision a dream world where everything is to our liking, the real world is just going to bring us down.

What we can try to do is to look for the things that we find good in the world and be thankful for them. Expect nothing, good or bad, and be pleasantly surprised when we do see something good.

All too often we see the advantages of others, especially others without a brain injury, and we become envious and believe that they have it easy; that they have it better than we do, and that just makes us miserable.

Everyone believes they have challenges. Everybody feels the tug of his or her responsibilities. Who are we to judge who has a harder row to hoe? Different things are harder for different people.

While it is very true that we have some added challenges, perhaps many added challenges, it is also true that we can have greater rewards. How many people get a feeling of accomplishment from tying their shoes? I happen to find that activity challenging. I always wear shoes with laces so that when I do get them on I can feel a certain self-satisfaction. I start each day with a victory.

Meditations

My point is that we have to appreciate the things that go right. These are not always obvious, but they are there. Seeing the good in life is a form of self-discipline. The news reports focus on the bad things in the world. So much of our recovery focuses on what is wrong. We need to reorient our worldview.

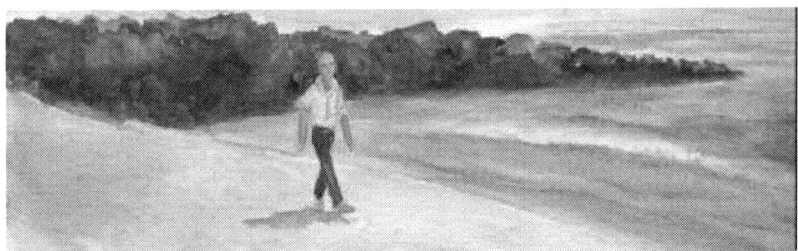

We need to believe in smiling. Why wait for a reason to smile? Why wait for something to make us smile, as though we are daring the world to even try? Let us smile pro-actively. We can grab the bull by the horns and smile when we realize that the bull's horns are in the shape of smile. Life can be very amusing. If we fill our lives with humor and compassion we will find that we don't have time for sadness.

Empower yourself, choose the mood you want and then create it. When we realize that we make a choice between sorrow and joy then we have no one else to blame if we are not joyful.

Mike Strand

Understanding Anger

I have heard people talk about the anger issues surrounding TBI. I have heard it said that TBI victims can have a terrible temper and that there is just no talking to them. It has been described as a symptom of TBI and that because of its organic nature there is nothing that can be done about it and that it is just a fact of life.

I see people shake their heads and say how unreasonable a TBI victim can be. Caregivers get frustrated. They wonder why the TBI victim can't (or won't) see that they are trying to help them. They feel that they are being taken for granted and are unappreciated. This is not true. Let me try to shed some light on what goes through a brain-injured mind.

When I am angry I believe that I am absolutely right and justified in being angry. The reasons that I am angry are as true to me as my feelings of anger. So often what a brain-injury means is being unable to communicate effectively. There are times when all the thoughts are clear in my head, but I just can't seem to get the words out. If I'm agitated it just gets worse.

When someone doesn't agree with those reasons, they usually try to explain the situation to me and say how I just am not taking certain things in consideration. What I "hear" is that I am wrong once again and have no business being angry. I still feel justified in my anger, I just feel like I am unable to explain myself clearly. In my effort to communicate more effectively I raise my voice and speak with more passion.

I give off more heat than light.

I also feel that if I were able to explain myself as clearly as I understand myself that they would suddenly

Meditations

understand my anger and the situation that is making me angry could finally be resolved.

It is very frustrating to see something wrong, terribly wrong, and be the only person able to see it that way. Oftentimes, the road I travel is so far removed from the road that other people travel that I can't possibly see things but in another way and from another angle.

People ask me if, after twelve years, I'm better. I tell them after twelve years it is easier for me to admit that perhaps a thing is not the way I see it; after twelve years I've learned that things are occasionally not as they seem to me.

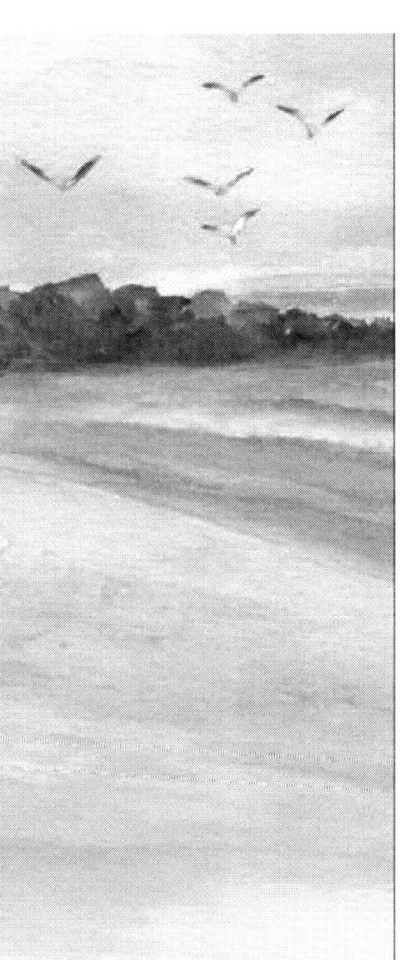

It has taken time for me to realize that just because I see something as square, it may not be square. It is just nice to hear that someone can see why I think it is square. They don't have to agree with me. They don't have to show me where I'm wrong. It's just nice to feel like I've been heard.

Otherwise, I'm angry and alone.

Mike Strand

Why Support Groups Are for You

I have run into a few people who have a brain injury but don't go to support groups because they have the idea that support groups are just for whiners and they don't whine and they don't want to listen to anyone else whine.

I agree with their sentiments about whining, but I believe they are mistaken in what they think a support group is. If support groups were just a bunch of whiners I wouldn't be involved in one.

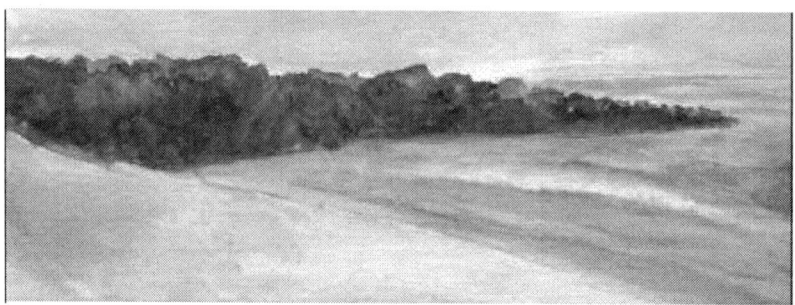

I go to a support group because *I don't like to whine.* In a support group they all know what I'm going through. I just have to say, "I was late for work because I took two showers in a row." Everyone there knows immediately how that feels and what it's like. If I tried to say that to ordinary people I would have to go through seemingly endless explanations that are fruitless and irritating.

I have found an unseen benefit to connecting with people at a support group. Since I feel like someone finally understands what I'm going through, I'm less inclined to talk to ordinary people about it.

Meditations

Talking to a non-survivor about my TBI just alienates them and makes them feel uncomfortable. They start avoiding me and soon I have no friends. By going to a support group I get that out of my system. My old friends begin to hang around me again. They admire my stoic courage in the face of adversity. They maybe can't say why, but now they enjoy my company much more.

So please, before you write off attending a support group, attend one and feel what it's like just to realize you are not alone.

Mike Strand

Without Crutches

Several years ago I met a young man with a brain injury. As often happens between fellow survivors, we became good friends. His accident had occurred when he was fourteen and he was then in his twenties. In spite of his many limitations he led an active lifestyle which primarily revolved around water sports at his parents lakefront cabin. Though he could not water-ski he enjoyed wake-boarding.

He walked with a four-point cane. His gate was slow and deliberate. When he went to sit down he would set his cane by the door and take his seat. As you might imagine, he was forever forgetting where he left his cane and would often have left it if he hadn't been so convinced he "needed" it to walk.

Watching him walk I noticed that it really didn't seem to matter whether or not he had his cane with him; he still had the same slow deliberate pace. One day I asked him why he used it and he told me it was because they gave it to him. I said that, in my opinion, as long as he used it he would always be dependent on it. This was not an educated opinion or a "positive thinking seminar" quote a la Dale Carnegie, it was just one friend speaking his mind.

The next time I saw him he had discarded his cane. A few years later when I saw him he was still walking without one. I'm not sure he was walking any better without it, but at least he didn't have to drag it around with him and wear it like a badge of infirmity (his words).

This episode illustrates a core belief of mine that government assistance programs can become crutches, they can institutionalize disability. Let me illustrate it another way.

Meditations

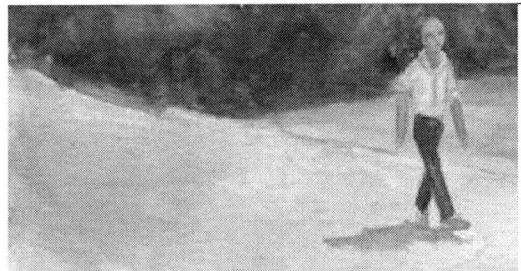

If a private company that manufactured crutches went around selling them to anyone they could convince needed them, in a very short time they would be accused of preying on a vulnerable population segment merely to make a profit.

On the other hand, if a government agency went around offering free crutches to anyone they could convince needed them, it would be called "serving the public."

It is important to realize that government programs are as dependent on consumers as for-profit companies. Their "profit" comes in the form of expanded budgets. This is why bureaucracies grow. No individual bureaucrat or aid worker is bad, but the whole public assistance bureaucracy is based on the flawed premise that greater public spending reduces want. Greater public spending creates want.

Which brings me back to my original point. Government programs need you to need them. You must judge for yourself what you need... what you really need, and when you've had enough.

I am not writing all this to argue a political agenda, though many will see it that way, I am addressing the survivors out there who are made dependent by programs that reward need and punish real recovery.

Mike Strand

Yoga

It is an established fact that the better physical shape you're in the better your recovery from traumatic brain injury is going to be. It not only helps your physical recovery it also helps your mental and emotional recovery as well.

The first thing you have to decide is what type of fitness is going to work well for you. Everyone is different and we all have different needs and desires. For me personally, I have chosen yoga. I tried many different activities and many of these I still enjoy doing, but yoga is the activity I would choose if I could only do one of them. Let me explain why I feel this way.

The first thing I want to address is flexibility. One of the most common comments regarding yoga is, "I can't do yoga, I'm horribly inflexible." This is not a reason to avoid yoga; it is a reason to do it. I was like everyone else when I started my yoga practice—I was stiff as a board. I'm much more flexible now than when I started, much more flexible than I would have ever thought possible. The unintended side effect of increased flexibility is the youthful feeling that it gives me.

The next thing I want to address is balance. Equilibrium was an aspect of my brain injury that continued to dog me even after I had overcome many other hurdles. My wife had tried a yoga class and suggested I might do the same because she thought it would help my balance. Boy was she right! The first few months of going three times a week didn't really produce tangible results, but I persevered and eventually I made some real progress. As I've said before, your balance is like a muscle, the more you use it the sharper it becomes. I'm still (after four years) not as stable as many yoga students, but I'm am dramatically ahead of where I was before.

Meditations

    Yoga is not competitive. You practice at a speed and skill that is right for you. Everyone's body and mind are different. What I noticed right away was that not only did I not compete with other people, I did not compete with that most implacable of all people, my former self. Since I had never done anything like yoga before I had no "old me" to compete against.

    You also gain strength and stamina. A lot of people say that they don't want to devote themselves totally to yoga because they want a more rounded work out. Yoga is an incredible strength training work out. When you get into some of these poses and try to hold them for ten or twenty seconds you will know what a real burn feels like. A simple technique that will give you an idea of what yoga feels like is this: open both your hands, spread your fingers as wide as you can and open your palm as far as possible. Hold it for ten seconds. Use all your strength. Remember to breathe. Breathing through the poses is so important, for strength, stamina, mental clarity, and discipline. Now make a fist with both hands. Squeeze as tight as you can. Hold for ten seconds. Remember to breathe. Now relax. Feel the energy in your hands. This is what yoga does for your whole body. Do you feel warmth? Now can you imagine how much of a workout yoga can be? Incidentally, this particular pose is an excellent exercise for anyone who is sitting at a desk all day, it really wakes you up and can help prevent Carpal Tunnel Syndrome.

    The best reason that I can think of for a TBI victim to practice yoga is what it does for the brain. Yoga means the union of mind and body. You begin yoga with a stiff body and an undisciplined mind and you work towards a limber body and a firm mind. Yoga tightens down all the loose screws in your head while acting like an oil can for the body. *Yoga puts me in control of my body, instead of me being a prisoner in my body.*

    If you would like to try yoga, I have a few suggestions. You may want to check out a few different places and find one that you feel comfortable with. Ask to talk to an instructor and see if they are responsive to your concerns and conditions. Once you find a place try it a few times. The first few times you may feel awkward. Stick it out! Go a few times and really give it a shot.

Mike Strand

If you feel that you can just sit back and pop all the right pills and get better, I feel sorry for you. It is necessary to take an active part in your recovery. It won't happen over night, but what have you got to lose?

What I really like about yoga is that it is not just about recovering what I had lost, it's about gaining a level of wellness that I have never known before. I can't compare myself to where I was before my accident because I'm already miles ahead. Imagine how good it feels to be able to say that. We all have that potential.

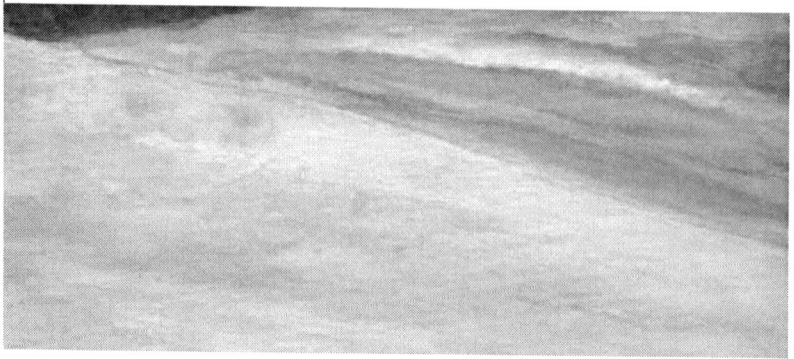

Meditations

A Near Horizon

One of the effects of a brain injury is what I call a near horizon. A horizon is the limit of one's perception. With a brain injury the ability to pick out details, especially key details, is severely limited.

This happens on many levels. Visual perception and even hearing are the most obvious because they are physical. Less apparent, but potentially more threatening are the difficulties of perceiving consequences and opportunities.

When I first began driving (about six months post injury) I thought I had tunnel vision. Yet, when I was tested, my vision was fine. What I realized some years later was that although my peripheral vision was fine, my brain's ability to process the full field of incoming visual images was seriously compromised. At a relatively quiet intersection I had little difficulty, but at a busy intersection it became, and still becomes, very challenging to sift through all the visual noise and select the valid images from the rest.

Looking for something makes me very uneasy.

Mike Strand

Whether I'm looking for a tool in the garage, or a salt shaker in the cupboard, or more often, my glasses. I find that if the item in question isn't right where I imagine it or if it doesn't look like I imagine it, then there is a good chance I won't see it.

Hearing is challenging because it requires concentration. A near by conversation in a restaurant or even a TV in an adjacent room can interfere with my ability to listen to what is being said directly to me. Add to that the open ended nature of human speech with its digressions and segues and an ordinary person can have trouble following along. Don't even get me started on disagreements with my significant other...

I'm sharing this so you don't think you're the only one. More often than not, if you're having a difficulty that ordinary people don't seem to have, or don't have to the extent you have, it probably is your brain injury.

How many times with brain injury do we have difficulty seizing up a situation that everybody else seems to know intuitively? Sometimes its as harmless as understanding a joke, sometimes it's as serious as not recognizing a swindle. How can you tell a good deal from one that's *too* good? This brain injury induced naivete can be quite a deficit. This is the number one reason that I don't feel confident that I could truly ever master independent living; Too many times my spouse has intervened and kept me from doing something, that in hindsight, was truly foolish.

Most often this perceptual difficulty is manifested by a lack of assertiveness. How can you be confident and assertive when you often times just don't know? When so many decisions seem completely arbitrary? On a consistent basis I am reminded by hindsight that I should have done this or I could have done that,

I have no pat answers. No pop psychology replies. I have no strategies to overcome these hurdles. Here I am fourteen years post accident, a relatively high functioning survivor, and these things are still before me. Oh well, life is worth what you pay for it.

Meditations

Sorrow to Wisdom

Sorrow is the path to wisdom. By turning sorrow into wisdom I can see a point to my pain. If I do not try to learn from my situation then I must admit my sorrow holds no meaning.

I don't view things as good or bad. Those are loaded terms that mean different things to different people. I view things as boring or interesting. One of my first thoughts that I can distinctly remember after coming out of my coma and learning what happened to me was "this is interesting." It wasn't "good" interesting or "bad" interesting. It was just interesting. As the wizard Gandalf said in *The Fellowship of the Ring,* "Even the very wise cannot see all ends." I have lived through many hardships, overcome a few hurdles, and fell over a few others. I am glad to have made the trip. A thing is worth what you are willing to pay for it. That which I have paid for dearly on a personal level I now prize highly. Real wisdom is never obtained easily.

Wisdom, like perfection, is not a goal to reach, but a point to move towards. There is not always a clear lesson to be learned from any tragedy, and besides, the lesson will be different for each individual. Richard Bach wrote that 'there is no such thing as a problem without a gift for you in its hands…You seek problems because you need their gifts.'

You may be saying, "Whoa, wait a minute Mike, I didn't seek a brain injury." That may be true, but fixing the blame on anyone but oneself is the path of a victim. It does not matter whose fault it was, it is my responsibility to heal and grow. I find it empowering to take responsibility for my accident; it gives me a feeling of control and independence. Those are two things that I often find in short supply with a brain injury.

Mike Strand

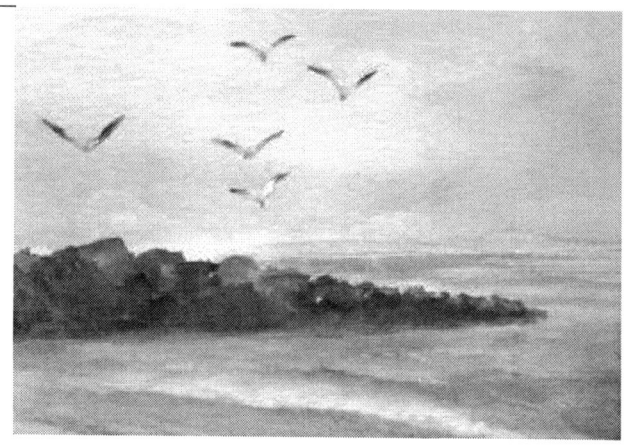

I must make one further comment on wisdom. Wisdom is not cynicism. A cynic views all things in the worst possible light: i.e., Murphy's Law. Cynicism is false wisdom. It destroys possibilities and it abandons reason. Things are not always bad. Reality is often a self-fulfilling prophecy, so one had better choose one's realities carefully.

Sorrow is part of a full life. Often, I hear TBI victims talking in positive terms and I wonder if it from having accepted their sorrow or having denied it. It is okay to be sad and angry after brain injury, it is even necessary. Let the emotion wash over you, fill you, even become you, and then watch it fade away. Eventually you do just get tired of being sad and angry, and that is the time to say goodbye to your sorrow and move on. Move on before your sorrow becomes your identity. You want to be able to say, "that was me being sorrowful, this is me having moved on."

Meditations

A Borrowed Identity

    A vague impression of my pre-TBI life. Remembrance of a past and an ID that is no longer me. I'm living on borrowed memory – A life lived by someone else. I don't remember it directly, but I can remember remembering. Like when you can remember a time when you knew all of your first grade classmate's names. You can remember when you could, but you cannot remember them now. Yes, it's like that, except now your whole past life is like that.

    If experiences shape our personas, and experiences are memories, aren't all memories valid whether or not others share them? I re-invent myself by cobbling memories together, yet it is difficult to assemble the past. I assemble my faint impressions into what I hope is a mosaic of my past life. Is this a fool's errand? Nobody remembers the same event in the same way. This makes trying to remember something problematic at best. Did something actually happen or not? Am I just imagining it? At what point does a memory of an event become fantasy? At what point exactly? How many errors are allowed before the image in my mind is no longer valid?

    Nobody remembers something the same. I am constantly reminded by others of things I did or said. All of these recollections could be factual...and different. Who, if anybody, is right?

    Our minds create memories to fill in gaps where we have no memory. When a person is missing as much memory as I am, then a lot of memory gets created. When a lot of my past is only in my mind, and the sum of who I am is my past, who am I?

    Sometimes these questions overwhelm me, much as they may have overwhelmed you as you read them just now.

Mike Strand

If this isn't an identity crisis, I don't know what is. As a survivor I have two identities, my pre-TBI and post-TBI self. They are not the same person and they don't really live in the same body. My ghost often haunts me, or should I say I often haunt my present self. The pre-TBI me is watching the post-TBI me trying to get through the day.

This isn't schizophrenia. This is a past life living in the present with me. Except, of course, I have all this baggage from my past life that I have brought into my present life. My relationships, my debts, my obligations, my things, my friends, the list goes on. Much of it I would not have chosen, much of it I would not give up. I must take it all. I try to continue on many of the same paths that the pre-TBI me was on before; it isn't always comfortable, nor is it ever easy, but changing it is even more uncomfortable and difficult. It would be much simpler to live in an apartment (why do they call them apartments when they are all together?) than in my house—I could just call the landlord if something didn't work instead of having to fix it myself—but I'm not going to sell my house and move into an apartment.

I don't consider myself lucky to be alive, that would mean being lucky to have a brain injury. The fact is I am alive and I have a brain injury. Luck is irrelevant. I play the hand I'm dealt. I am choosing the best possible life. Long ago, before my brain-injury, I told myself that if I wasn't actually being shot at things were all right. Now and again I have to remind myself to relax, at least I'm not being shot at.

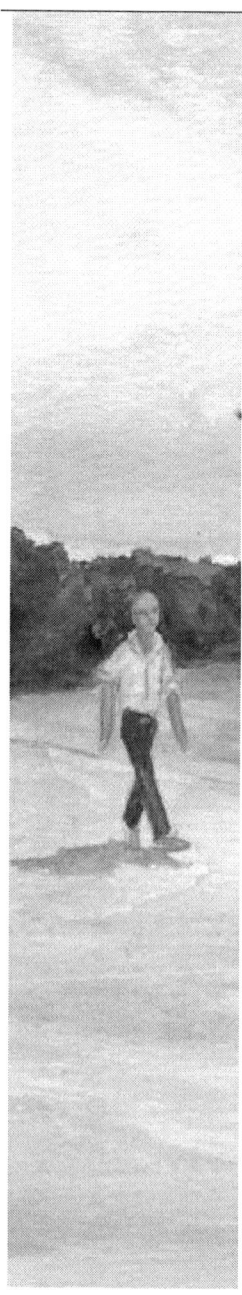

Meditations

So I move on. I do the life thing and I am generally happy, but every so often I question who I am. Every day I'm building the new me, but what is my foundation? Letting go of one's past is very difficult and having one's past torn away isn't any easier. The Czechoslovakian writer Milan Kundera writes about "the unbearable lightness of being" where someone lets go of all things familiar and just lives in the moment. He maintains that most people find that kind of life, a life devoid of reference and familiarity, to be a life without reassurance and comfort. Welcome to my world. These are the demons I struggle with when I am tired and overwhelmed. This is when my pre-TBI self looks at my post-TBI self and says, "man, it sure sucks to be you."

It is times like this when I must turn to strengths, like my yoga and my sense of humor, and it is also when I need to admit that I'm tired and that I really must get some sleep.

Mike Strand

How Others See You

It's so hard trying to imagine what others must think of us. We know they think we're different now. They marginalize us; somehow what we think isn't as valid as it was before.

Oftentimes this is grounded in some very good reasoning. We have difficulty expressing ourselves. We forget what we were saying right in mid-sentence. If we are interrupted we can become totally lost as we lose our train of thought.

All this leads to our own insecurities. We know we get confused. Even ordinary folks feel insecure about what others think about them, especially if they are having an off day. Well, we are having an off life. Naturally we are going to wonder how others perceive us.

All this insecurity can lead to massive problems in our interpersonal relationships. Again, we feel alone and shut off. Isolated. We close ourselves off to others, and now our inability to communicate is further increased by our unwillingness to risk exposure to censure.

I've been calling this insecurity, but I feel quite secure. I am certain that many times I sound like an idiot and that I say stupid things. I know when I say something, very often, it was not what I intended to say, and that I missed making my point. This confidence in my own fallibility is what bothers me. Surely others are as aware of it and as unforgiving as I am.

Is this all in our mind? What to do? If you say nothing your brain will lead you astray. For example, you know how your memory fills in gaps, until you begin remembering things that didn't actually happen. The same is true for how people feel about you. Unless something is said, your brain

Meditations

begins constructing how you think they probably feel about you. Then, based on how you think they feel about you, you begin to filter their words and actions through these assumptions, and it snowballs. This is the general outline of many sitcoms where failure to communicate leads to all

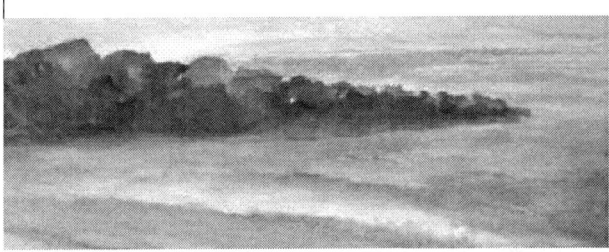

sorts of zany scenarios. But people play life more seriously and there is no writer to put in a happy ending (when the truth comes out and everyone just dismisses the happenstance with a polite news-anchor chuckle). This is life and there is no 30-minute resolution.

Given this situation, what can a survivor do? How can we be proactive and not reactive? Here is a strategy that works for me:

Ask them how they feel. Reflect your thoughts on them. "Do you feel I'm less competent now?" They will probably tell you no. They may actually have been thinking exactly that (you are less competent), but now that you are asking them directly they will go out of their way to show you that they don't feel that way about you. Being social creatures we tend to behave the way we're treated. They treat us like competent people and we become confident in our own competence.

It doesn't really matter what they actually thought. Imagine if what you thought about somebody were immediately broadcast to them. Polite civil behavior reminds us to be kind. You don't have to lie. You don't have to call someone fat, even if that's what you're thinking. If your brain injury prevents you from filtering out your comments, then you know how much trouble and needless pain *that* can cause.

They may actually tell you how and in what way they do feel about you. This is good, even if you are not happy to hear what they have to say – at least now you know how you come off. Try not to be defensive. I know this is perhaps the hardest thing in the world, especially about your brain injury, but view their honesty as a gift. It is a useful tool you can use to improve yourself.

If they say you have certain faults (no doubt you are aware of your faults, we all are), what you can say is, "I'm working really hard at overcoming these things. Can you help me to be a better person?" Obviously, you are probably not going to say exactly that but you can get the gist I'm driving at.

Communicating is always better than not.